Stress

By:

Dr. Chidozie J. Ononuju
DO, Pharm D, PhD

ISBN: 978-1530903146
         1530903149
LCCN: 2016905812

Table of Contents

Table of Contents (continued)

Forward

Stress is a normal human reaction to pressure. As a medical student (many years ago) stress was almost regarded as a necessary measure when studying medicine. Long nights and early mornings resulted in a stressful time in my life. Some stress is good though. I remember the birth of my first son. I was anxious, nervous and finally when he was born, relieved that everything went as planned.

There is no doubt that the body goes through physiological changes when enduring any type of stress (good or bad) but as a medical doctor I have seen numerous patients with chronic illnesses and otherwise who experienced those illnesses due to overwhelming stress. Money problems, relationship problems, grief, work deadlines, etc. I could go on and on. Stress is real thing and in this fast paced society where technology was meant to simplify our lives, many of us are overworked and unaware of our body's needs.

I have given many patients the prescription for "rest" but I am sure that over half of them did not do it. I know this because their body indicated in subsequent visits that they did not. I didn't write this book to scare anyone but rather to make aware of the dangers of stress and its counterparts like anxiety, depression, cancer, premature aging, chronic illnesses and so on.

Read through and evaluate your life chapter by chapter conceptualizing each thought and asking yourself the following questions; do I desire to live a long life, do I strive to be healthy, do I often take time to do things I enjoy, am I getting enough sleep, am I getting enough daily exercise, are my goals in life prioritized...

No one realistically can answer "yes" to all of these questions simultaneously but the goal is to get you thinking about these things. The more aware you are the least likely you are to totally ignore stress.

Acknowledgements

This book is dedicated to my wife Gloria Ononuju who supports me in all I do, my mother Cordelia Ononuju and late grandmother Uredia Nwache who were always my inspirations. To my favorite uncle, mentor and teacher Mr. Eugene Ijeoma Ononuju who guided my education in the United States and whom I regard as the pillar of my success.

Chapter One

Stress in America

Stress has many definitions in both medical and psychological terms. Stress is also viewed by individuals, societies and cultures differently. Merriam-Webster defines stress as "a state of mental tension and worry caused by problems in your life, work, etc., or something that causes strong feelings of worry or anxiety: physical force or pressure". How you look at stress may be significantly different than how someone else views stress in their own life. We all have different values and different lifestyles so stress affects individuals differently. Everyone experiences stress in their lives at some point or another. How you deal with stress and your ability to cope are very important in whether or not the stress will affect you mentally and physically. To sum it up easily, stress is your body's response to events that interrupt your normal life and daily living.

In order to provide a holistic picture of stress and how it affects people, culture and daily living vary in different groups of people. For example, Minorities such as Blacks and Hispanics may have different stressors in living and work environments that Whites may not have. Racial disparities in health are evident to most physicians that see patients regularly. According to American Psychological Association, Minority health overall is worse than Whites. Viewing stress from a multicultural perspective is important in order to create specific ways of coping and eliminating stress. Middle class in Americans strive to make more money and enjoy luxuries from life. Modern psychologists are now learning the importance of viewing stress through a multi-cultural lens instead of historically viewing stress from a Euro- American perspective.

Familiar Stress

We all experience stress in our daily lives. Everyone deals with pressures and daily demands of making a living and supporting themselves or their families. American society has a high stress culture that places importance on money. American lifestyles are success driven and this causes people to work to support their spending habits and day to day living expenses. If you have nice things like a home, car and expensive possessions in America you are considered "successful". Most people in America want some sort of comfort and work life balance in their lives like vacation and travel, luxury vehicles, homes and entertainment.

In order to maintain or enjoy these nice things, one may have to work hard in order to pay for those things. Working hard for some involves stress and anxiety to keep up with their lifestyle and debt. American society is divided by classes, the wealthy, the middle class and the poor. The class system is important to remember when it comes to coping with stress and pressure. The poor and the middle class experience more stress due to lack of money and resources. The wealthy class may not have the pressures and demands of stress like the middle class and poor because they possess money, resources and capital. Research shows that over the years, the middle class is shrinking and there is a wider gap growing between the rich and the poor classes. America is made up of many different ethnicities.

Ethnically, we all handle stress differently. We will discuss Caucasian, African American and Hispanic cultures and how stress affects them differently. Minorities are at greater risk for disease more than Whites in America. Minorities may deal with different factors of stress, environment and health issues than Caucasians or Whites.

It is important to understand how the difference in culture affects how we all deal with stress. According to the Center for Disease Control, African American, American Indian and Hispanic women have the highest risk for becoming overweight. Asian Americans have a lower obesity rate than the general population. This could mean that minority women are more prone to stress more than Caucasians due to different levels of education, access to healthcare and proper nutrition. Obesity is at an epidemic high and there are several diseases that stem from obesity such as heart disease, cancer, stroke and diabetes.

Many situations can cause stress. Some people experience stress from their jobs or work, from raising children, paying bills, or even dealing with difficult spouses or family members. The American Psychological Association conducts research every year on stress in America, according to the 2013 report, the first cause of stress is Money, next is work and then the last cause is the economy. Some stress may not be all bad like starting a new job or studying for an exam at school, but it still puts the mind and body under pressure and affects you in some way.

Stress affects your body mentally and/ or physically. That means that you are going to experience symptoms in your body or in your mind that can affect your mental state. It is also important to remember that in most cases, our bodies and minds have two responses to stress: fight or flight. How you deal with stress is important for you to learn so you can take care of yourself mentally and physically. Stress for long periods of time can damage parts of your body like your brain, nerves, muscles, joints, heart, stomach, and the reproductive system. Prolonged periods of stress on the body can contribute to diseases like depression, heart disease and high blood pressure. According to American Psychological Association, 61% of adults say that managing stress is extremely or very important, but only 35% say they are doing an excellent or very good job at it. Managing stress in healthy ways is important for everyone to know to live healthier lives and to feeling

better.

Chapter Two

Ethnic probabilities of stress

African Americans and Stress

Research has shown that Blacks are exposed to more poverty, crime, substance abuse than Whites. African-Americans culturally, may be exposed to different stress factors due to their environments, family upbringing and economic status. Blacks may suffer more discrimination and harassment in school, work and everyday living. This puts them at risk for chronic stress and more exposure to illness, disease and even death. One study found that Blacks have more pressure to outperform their colleagues due to discrimination in the workplace and feel the need to prove their work ethic which places more demands and stress on their work lives.

Due to many factors, Blacks face more high stress situations that may lead to implications of health both psychically and mentally. Black men face high amounts of stressors due to their role in society and their respective families. Culturally, the man faces economic pressures of providing for his family and even can be the sole provider of his parents due to economic conditions. Culturally, racial discrimination and profiling is a reality with Black men. Black men also are culturally and socially conditioned to be strong and to not show emotions or vulnerability, this causes men to view taking care of themselves as a sign of weakness.

According to some health statistics, Black men are less likely to seek regular health check-ups and routine visits which place them at greater risk of not being properly diagnosed with several health issues like hypertension and high cholesterol.

According to an article published in the Los Angeles Times, statistics show that Black men have a shorter life expectancy than any other race group in America except Native Americans. This means that the state of health in Black men in America is a very alarming issue that should be addressed by our nation. They also have a shorter life expectancy than African American women. There may be many reasons for this such as lifestyle, nutrition, healthcare and exercise. Another issue may be the way men and women deal with emotional and physical stress very differently.

Black women culturally are nurturers and caregivers in the family and face many stressors from multiple caregiving roles at home and work. Culturally, Black women believe in being strong, supportive and taking care of their men and children. They often place value and importance on ensuring everyone is taken care of at their expense and health. A study in 2010 published by CDC also states the first cause of death in women is heart disease. Black women are leading in heart disease over Hispanics and Whites. The second leading cause of death is cancer. Finally, the third cause of death in black women is stroke.

Hispanics and Stress

Stressors of poverty, discrimination, acculturation, immigration and environment are evident in Hispanic culture very similar to African-American culture. Hispanics rely heavily on family and community to assist in times of crisis or stress, unfortunately due to their dependence on their relationships to solve problems, mental health issues such as depression and substance abuse go undetected and untreated. According to American Psychiatric Association, Latinos have been shown to suffer from mental illnesses or emotional disturbances at a higher rate than other groups. The study also showed that the Hispanic population uses mental health services less than other ethnic groups. Hispanic men culturally view themselves as brave, strong and are often labeled "Machismo" in their family and work roles. The stressors in Hispanic men are lack of information, language barriers, and cultural values that lead them to feel they should solve their own problems. These cultural stressors lead to higher instances of depression and alcohol abuse in Hispanic men according to a study by Diane Hales, however fewer enter treatment. The National Alliance on Mental Illness indicates that depression in Hispanics occurs at a higher rate than other ethnicities and states they are at higher risk for mental illness, anxiety and substance abuse.

Hispanic women have similar stressors as African-American women such as being the nurturer and caregiver of multiple family members, poverty, and experience more barriers with the added pressures of acculturation. Hispanic women are leading #2 for Cancer cause of death. Hispanic women also tend to experience depression and issues with mental illness over other ethnicities.

Whites and Stress

Whites experience stress but most studies and research shows that overall, the risk factors for disease and mortality are higher for minority groups, such as Blacks and Hispanics. Whites have different ways of coping and dealing with stress and anxiety than minorities. According to the U. S. Department of Health and Human Services, a study reported that whites receive more mental health services and treatment and have more access to mental health care. Culturally, it is acceptable and a norm for whites to seek therapy when in crisis or going through life hardships such as divorce, loss of loved one or a job loss. Whites traditionally, do not deal with the same stressors that minorities deal with such as lower socio-economic status, discrimination, environmental, and educational barriers. Culturally, whites both men and women view getting help or talking out their problems or seeking assistance as healthy and taking care of themselves.

Whites handle relationship problems, work issues and family crisis differently because of social conditioning and cultural upbringing. A study about differences in ethnicities in coping with stress revealed that white women find stress relief by devoting more time to their children and seeking support from friends. Black women in this same study tended to children and sought friendly support as well but avoided problems from others. Men in this study both Black and Whites confronted whatever or whoever was causing the stress or just removed themselves from the situation. Economically, whites earn more than more and have a higher net worth than minorities. This could indicate that whites are not exposed to as much stress such as job strain, low status, environmental hazards, neighborhood instability, poverty, and physical deprivation. Traditionally, whites also seek the assistance of professionals when caring for a parent or an ill spouse. They have access to more resources such as nursing homes and health care while minorities may suffer the burden of care for families and spouses which causes greater stress and financial hardship.

There are many cultural and social differences that affect the ways different groups cope with stress, however the fact still remains that there are clear differences in stressors and the exposure to stressful situations for different groups to consider. This is an important part of looking at how and why we deal with stress in comparison to others. Disease and illness from stress is a global issue and should be viewed from a world perspective in order to minimize health risks and the mortality rate.

Chapter Three

Recognizing Stress

It is important to recognize stress or take measures to eliminate stress as much as possible to avoid further problems. How does one recognize stress? What are some symptoms and revealing signs of stress? Taking inventory of stress begins by asking a series of questions and assessing how one feels mentally and physically. Stress affects the mind, emotions and the body (thoughts, feelings and behavior). There are several online tools to determine stress, as well as helpful information to assist in managing stress. Some questions to ask to help identify stressors are:

1) How often do I experience headaches? Do I have chest pain?
2) Am I often tense, sore or do I often experience pain in my body?

3) Am I experiencing stomach problems?

4) Am I often tired, fatigued or restless? Am I experiencing sleep problems?

5) Has there been a change in my sex drive?

6) Am I anxious, irritable, angry, sad or depressed?

7) Am I overeating or under eating?

8) Am I using abusing alcohol, tobacco, or other drugs?

9) Do I have angry outbursts, easily frustrated and lose my focus often?

10) Am I withdrawing socially and not motivated?

Asking all of these questions honestly

and noting the frequency is important because

these questions will help to discern the
thoughts, emotions and behaviors that result
from stress. It also may be helpful to journal
stress or stressful thoughts to determine the
frequency and intervals of stressful situations in
daily living. If one is dealing with illnesses such
as heart disease, high blood pressure, diabetes,
cancer or other illnesses, these symptoms should
be taken seriously and monitored by a
physician. If the answer to most of these
questions is yes, it may be time to talk to a
physician or create a plan to eliminate issues
causing stress on the body and mind. Early
recognition is better so that one can manage
stress before stress overload.

Types of Stress

The two main types of stress are acute stress and chronic stress. Acute stress is when the initial response the body has to threatening situations; this is the reaction of "fight or flight" which is sometimes the body's own way of protecting from immediate danger like avoiding a crash or accident. Acute stress normally does not cause major issues because once the perceived threat is gone, the body returns to its normal state. Acute stress only begins to cause problems when it is very frequent and regular, for example panic attacks or Post-traumatic stress disorder (PTSD).

Chronic stress is developed through a series of acute stress instances that never go away. The body's fight or flight response is no longer being used to this type of stress because chronic stress builds over time and causes more problems and the effects may sometimes be long-term. A study conducted by the American Psychological Association (2013) reported a link of chronic stress to obesity, depression and heart disease.

Merriam-Webster defines a stressor as "something that makes your worried or anxious: a source of stress, a stimulus that causes stress".

There are two types of stressors:

➢ Internal- inside

➢ External- outside

This indicates stressors can be categorized by things that are within one's span of control (easy to manage) or out of one's span of control (more difficult to manage). Inside stressors are often within our control or may be self-induced and can sometimes develop from external stressors. Internal stressors caused by unhealthy thoughts, behaviors and actions may be controlled or changed. External stressors are outside of one's ability to control or are from external factors in the environment and outer conditions. Moreover, stress is coming from inside you or outside of you and most of the

time you have the ability to control and manage

both to maintain balance and health.

Internal Stressors

Earlier it was stated that often stress for individuals is often what is perceived or believed about a particular event circumstances. It is often the meaning given to a situation or the response we choose to have toward a situation that causes it to be stressful. What are some examples of internal stressors? Internal stressors for some may be:

➢ Negative self-talk (pessimism)

➢ Rigidity

➢ Expectations

➢ Limiting beliefs

➢ Low self esteem

- ➢ Misperceptions

- ➢ Attitude

- ➢ People pleasing

- ➢ Perfectionism

- ➢ Personality

Internal stress is often caused from within us, particularly from inside our mind by the thoughts we think which affect our moods, feelings, and attitudes. Stress often develops from internalizing external factors and not managing those factors in healthy ways or seeking support. This kind of internal stress is self-imposed by having self-defeating thoughts or unrealistic expectations of ourselves.

Thoughts of worry, negative self-talk (past programming), perfectionism and fear causes anxious feelings or a negative attitude. All of these internal thoughts, feelings and attitudes can cause emotional and physical symptoms to manifest if prolonged and not managed.

External Stressors

External stressors are environmental or real situations and circumstances that come from outside of us. Often, external stressors are not as easy to manage, for example an unfortunate incident outside of your control such as death or a sudden disability. What is important to be mindful of about external stressors is the management of stress and utilizing techniques that will assist in dealing with situations and lessen the stress. Unhealthy habits or inappropriate management of external events can lead to internal stressors and chronic stress.

Some examples of external stressors are:

➤ Major life events/changes

➤ Workplace conditions/challenges

➤ Relationships/divorce

➤ Income or financial difficulties

➤ Unsafe living environment

➤ Injury/trauma

➤ Children/family

➤ Death/loss

➤ Health issues

➤ Environmental or social factors Sometimes

   external factors are not just single events and

situations, often more than one event is present in daily life with another and it can become overwhelming and cause one to feel like they have no control due to pressure. It is important to identify solutions to change conditions if possible, it is also important to seek support to manage issues to keep from overload.

There are many different signs and symptoms of stress, the importance is to detect stressors early and know the triggers which may vary for different individuals. When the automobile "check engine" light comes on, this is often a warning to prevent damage to the vehicle and get it checked out.

Think of the body as a vehicle that needs regular maintenance and heed the warning signs that something needs to be changed, investigated or repaired when dealing with stress. Often the body sends physical signals when stressed out or under pressure such as headaches, stomach upset, tension in neck and shoulders, excessive worry, anxious feelings, sleep trouble, or appetite changes just to name a few. This is the body's way of sending signals or warning that attention or a change is needed. When ignored or not attended, symptoms may worsen such as depression, anxiety disorders and disease.

It is important to become self-aware and do an assessment in order to recognize what triggers will cause one to experience stress and furthermore, to understand how to manage the responses to triggers.

Here are some warning signs:

➢ Inability to focus and concentrate

➢ Moodiness or extreme irritability

➢ Feeling lost or unusually sad

➢ Emotional highs and lows (unstable)

➢ Unable to make decisions, frequent frustration

➢ Overwhelmed, extreme pressure

➢ Oversleeping or under sleeping

➢ Less energy or apathy

➢ Change in eating habits

➢ Using tobacco or alcohol to relieve
tension or stress

Stress Management

Stress management is about selfawareness, knowing what your sources of stress are, and creating strategies to cope or manage them effectively. Many of these strategies will involve changing daily routines such as diet, sleep, exercise, and relaxation. To maintain a healthy balance, this may require seeking medical help, creating a strong support system and learning new techniques to manage work, family and self-care. According to the American Psychological Association (APA) in 2012, "only 37percent of Americans feel they are actually doing an excellent or very good job of managing their stress."

It is important to remember that stress is subjective and what may be stressful for one individual may not be stressful to someone else, the same applies to stress management. The key is to find what works best for your individual lifestyle and preference. Awareness and recognition of stress symptoms is important so that stressors can be identified and managed. Even small steps taken one day at a time can help to eliminate stress. Stress may be unavoidable completely, that is why healthy management is essential.

Chapter Four

Neurological Effects of Stress

From a neurological perspective, stress impairs learning and judgment by cell damage in the hippocampus which is a part of the brain required for learning and memory. When the brain is under stress, this may prevent memory storage. A research study conducted in 2008 by the University of California Irvine found that the stress hormone cortisol affects the neurons by damaging pathways. This disintegration of the neurons hinders the ability to store information and identify information. In other words, the part of the brain that assists with memory and reasoning is hindered by acute stress. When a person's reasoning is affected, the ability to make good decisions and use sound judgment is impaired. This happens for several reasons, your ability to think clear and focus is clouded by stress and how it is currently affecting you. Sometimes under extreme pressure, the consequences of a decision may not be carefully weighted out if one wasn't under worry or pressure. Often snap judgments are made and one may overestimate the positive side of the current situation of the present moment and make permanent decisions that may have effects on the long term. Emotional decisions are common under stress and anxiety, often just to relive the stress of the moment. It is important to recognize that important decisions should be delayed until the stress is released.

The Central Nervous System (CNS) controls most functions of the body and mind. It consists of two parts: the brain and the spinal cord. The brain is the center of our thoughts, the interpreter of our external environment, and the origin of control over body movement. Stress affects how the Central Nervous System functions. There are two parts to the nervous system which are the central and peripheral. The central system is made up of the brain and spinal cord and the peripheral part is outside of the central nervous system that communicates information to and from the central nervous system and other parts of the body. Why is this important to know one might ask? Because the nerves in the peripheral system connect sensory organs such as muscles, eyes, ears, blood vessels and glands to the central system. There are several different nerve types, some do many functions such as regulate the heart muscles and the tiny muscles that line the walls of blood vessels and different glands. When triggered negatively, the CNS is affected negatively.

Emotional Stress

Emotional stress can affect your thoughts, your work and your relationships and harm your ability to function normally from day to day. Some symptoms of emotional stress can be overeating, under-eating, forgetfulness, crying spells, worry, fatigue or insomnia, irritability, anger or increased drinking or turning to substance abuse to cope. Emotional health is related to overall physical health. Eastern philosophy has embraced the effectiveness of positive emotional health and established practices to maintain emotional well-being and balance.

Western society is adopting this view although it is a slow process and the lower socioeconomic population and their cultural or religious beliefs may conflict with this philosophy. Overall mental health will improve overall physical health. Often obesity is related to physical health problems however, it is not treated as a mental issue. There are studies that link emotional health to physical health.

When under metal stress or anxiety, there is a reaction which happens in the body that cannot be seen or felt. It is important to understand what the body endures when it is under duress or distress.

Eustress

Eustress is the opposite of distress. The term eustress can be defined as good stress or positive emotions that are beneficial for wellbeing. This is the kind of feeling you get when you are experiencing joy, excitement and contentment. An example may be when you are excited about a goal you set and you finally accomplish that goal and you feel good feelings about yourself and finishing what you started. If people did not experience eustress, they wouldn't be productive or happy in life. Eustress prevents depression and promote neurological wellness within the body. Eustress makes distress easier to cope with.

Depression and Stress

The National Institute for Mental Health (NIMH) defines depression as a common but serious illness and states that most people who are depressed need treatment in order to get better. They define major depression as "severe symptoms that interfere with your ability to work, sleep, study, eat and enjoy life. An episode can occur only once in a person's lifetime, but more often, a person has several episodes". It is important to seek treatment for depression even if not major but mild to prevent future episodes. Some symptoms may not get treated due to not recognizing one is experiencing depression. Symptoms of depression may vary with individuals; however, here are some according to NIMH (2104):

- ➢ Persistent sad, anxious, or "empty" feelings.

- ➢ Feelings of hopelessness or pessimism.

- ➢ Irritability, restlessness, fatigue, decreased energy or insomnia.

- ➢ Loss of interest in activities or hobbies once pleasurable, including sex.

- ➢ Difficulty concentrating, remembering details, and making decisions.

- ➢ Overeating or appetite loss.

- ➢ Thoughts of suicide, attempts.

> Aches or pains, headaches, cramps, or digestive problems that do not ease even with treatment.

According to the Center for Disease Control, a 2006-2008 survey found that 1 in 10 adults reported depression. This study also revealed that the following groups meet the defined criteria for depression:

> Persons 45-64 years of age

> Women

> Blacks, Hispanics, non-Hispanic persons of other races or multiple races

> Persons with less than a high school education

> Those previously married

> Individuals unable to work or unemployed

> People without health insurance coverage

Being properly diagnosed and treated for depression is important especially when under chronic stress. There is a strong link between stress and depression which is due to the stress hormone cortisol. The body's response to prolonged stress can cause over-activity of the stress response mechanism (fight or flight) and affect the neurological system. This over-activity can deter normal body processes to function or maintain homeostasis.

Anxiety Disorders and Stress

Anxiety is a normal emotion that one experiences in life, for example, one may feel anxious before a big meeting at work or before giving birth to a child. These are expected, normal responses to situations, however, anxiety disorders and panic attacks are different that common anxiety and emotions. The Anxiety and Depression Association of America (AADA) defines a panic attack as "the abrupt onset of intense fear or discomfort that reaches a peak within minutes and includes at least four of the following symptoms:

➢ Palpitations, pounding heart, or accelerated heart rate.

- Sweating.

- Trembling and shaking.

- Sensations of shortness of breath or smothering.

- Feelings of choking.

- Chest pain and discomfort.

- Nausea or abdominal distress.

- Feeling dizzy, light-headed or faint.

- Chills or heat sensations.

- Paresthesia (numbness or tingling sensations)

- De- realization (feelings of unreality) or depersonalization (being detached from oneself)

➤ Fear of losing control or "going crazy" ➤ Fear of dying

It is important to seek medical attention with any of these symptoms due to some of these being similar to other physical problems like heart disease or thyroid issues. Panic attacks are strongly related to stress and anxiety disorders.

There are several types of anxiety disorders; Obsessive Compulsive Disorder (OCD), Post Trauma Stress Disorder (PTSD), and General Anxiety Disorder (GAD) to name a few. The AADA (2014) defines Generalized Anxiety Disorder (GAD) as "persistent, excessive, and unrealistic worry about everyday things". GAD affects over 6 million adults in the U.S. a year

and women are twice likely to be affected.

Symptoms of GAD are as follows:

> Constant worry, fear and pessimism.

> Muscle tension.

> Fatigue, restlessness and difficulty
sleeping

People with GAD are often burdened with

worry over unsubstantiated issues and it

sometimes occurs throughout the whole day

making it difficult to function through normal

social activities like family, work and school.

Both panic attacks and anxiety disorders have

various methods of treatment if diagnosed

properly, therapy and medical treatment is recommended for both, however cognitive behavioral therapy has been found to be a successful and helpful treatment to assist in changing the thinking errors and patterns that cause the worry and anxiety from both.

Here are several tips and strategies by ADAA (2014) to manage or minimize panic, anxiety and stress:

- ➤ Take a "time-out". Practice relaxation techniques such as; yoga, listen to music, meditate or get a massage.

- ➤ Stepping back from the problem helps clear your head.

- ➤ Eat well-balanced meals. Do not skip any meals.

- ➤ Limit alcohol and caffeine

- Get enough sleep.

- Exercise daily.

- Take deep breaths. Inhale and exhale slowly.

- Count to 10 slowly.

- Do your best. Instead of aiming for perfection.

- Accept that you cannot control everything.

- Welcome humor.

- Maintain a positive attitude.

Chapter Five

Aging & Sleep

Recent research has linked premature aging with stress and anxiety. As discussed earlier, stress causes systems in the body to slow function or limit functions which in turn, leaves one more susceptible to disease and illness. According to the American Institute of Stress, our immune system's defense mechanisms changes and the ability for the body to ward off infection declines. The immune system's response to chronic stress may accelerate the aging process and is related to the body's response to hidden inflammation. The Institute conducted a study in 2012 on telomere research and found a connection between shorter telomeres and anxiety. The research found that women who suffered from "phobic anxiety"

had shorter telomeres. Telomeres are protective

sections of DNA on the ends of chromosomes;

the length of telomeres can be helpful about cell

aging. Scientists have linked shorter telomeres

to cancers, heart diseases, dementia and other

diseases according to the Medical Daily Journal

(2012).

Aging at a Cellular Level

People may ask the question, why do we age or what causes one to grow old? Many researchers have different theories. Physiologically, the process of aging occurs as a result of damage to the cells in the body. The molecules in the cells such as DNA and RNA (proteins, nucleic acids and lipids) become damaged or mutated by many different internal and external causes. These causes are believed to be from wear and tear on the body over time. Think of how a vehicle works, when it is brand new, all the systems and options work great, however, in time, maintenance is needed and the car breaks down with time. The body when young and growing works similar to a new vehicle, the immune system, neural and endocrine systems are working properly. As one grows older, cell degeneration occurs from changes in body weight, metabolism, (lean body mass) and loss of tissues.

The body's physical process of aging involves the changing of cells, they function less efficiently and the organ's functionality. These cell changes cause many of the systems such as the muscular system, nervous system and the immune system to function differently. Cells divide a limited number of times, telomeres limit cell division and become shorter and shorter until eventual damage or cell death. As the body ages, changes in appearance take place

and the capability of an organ to function

normally changes as well. Physical changes to

vision, bone density and memory are just a few

that are associated with aging.

Stress and Sleep

An important part of health and well-being is sleep and getting plenty of rest for the body to function properly. The National Sleep Foundation conducted a study in 2005 and found that sleep requirements vary within age groups and that the amount of sleep an individual needs varies based on lifestyle and productivity. While some may feel healthy, productive and happy with seven hours of sleep, others may need nine to feel like they are functioning their best. People that have health issues such as obesity and other illnesses may require more sleep than someone who is healthy; therefore the rule of thumb for number of hours of sleep will require one to consider health, lifestyle and how they feel with the amount of sleep they are getting each night.

Sleep may also be negatively affected by stress and various situational factors. Some individuals may get less sleep or not enough sleep, a condition commonly referred to insomnia. Fatigue happens when individuals sleep too much or oversleep. Both insomnia and fatigue may have adverse effects on the body, and both may affect long term physical and mental health. Lack of sleep or insomnia may be caused by physiological health factors or psychological factors according to research. It is important to note that The National Sleep Foundation (2014) research shows that lack of sleep may have negative health outcomes such as:

> Increased risk of drowsy driving

> Increase of body mass index – a greater likelihood of obesity due to an increased appetite caused by sleep deprivation

> Increased risk of diabetes and heart problems

> Increased risk for psychiatric conditions including depression and substance abuse

> Decreased ability to pay attention, react to signals or remember new information

Stress and anxiety are the most common psychological causes of insomnia and fatigue. Depression is strongly associated with insomnia and fatigue and can worsen symptoms and further complicate sleep habits.

Some tips to help one with insomnia get more rest for positive mental health are:

> Maintain a regular sleep schedule and designate times.

> Eat healthy and limit caffeine, alcohol and eliminate smoking.

> Adjust room temperature ensuring comfortability and darken the room.

> Do soothing activities before bedtime such as bathing, reading or listening to soft music; avoid

stimulating activities like television and electronics such as cell phones and computers.

➢ Record daily habits and routines for awareness.

Chapter Six

Cancer

The National Cancer Institute defines cancer as "diseases in which abnormal cells divide without control and invade other tissues, cancer cells can spread to other parts of the body through the blood and lymph systems". There are many types of cancer, depending on what organ or cell type they originate in will determine the name of the cancer. Some examples of types of cancer are:

➢ Leukemia- cancer in blood forming tissues such as bone marrow that causes many abnormal blood cells to be produced and enter the blood stream.

➢ Central Nervous System Cancers- cancers that start in the brain and spinal cord tissues.

➢ Lung Cancer (cancer that begins in the lungs).

➢ Lymphoma and Myeloma- cancer that begins in the cells of the immune system.

➢ Breast Cancer- cancer that starts in the breast tissues.

It is important to understand that there are different types of cancer, however all cancer begins in the cells which is our body's basic make-up. The body's cells function in a way that divide and produce more cells to maintain health. When the cells divide abnormally or genetic material such as DNA become damaged, mutations of cells may produce disorder of growth and improper division. When our body's healthy cells die or are damaged, new healthy cells are produced; cancer is the disorder of this process. The extra cells produced may form a collection or a mass known as a tumor. Tumors may be benign (non-cancerous) can be removed, malignant (cancerous) tumors invade tissue and spread.

Treatment for cancer is available, the importance of detecting cancer early by scheduling regular visits with physician, proper diet, avoiding cancer risk factors and appropriate treatment cannot be underestimated. Early detection is critical to health and survival. More helpful information can be located at cancer.gov or the National Cancer Institute.

The body's response to stress is negatively related to creating habits that may increase risks for cancer such as smoking, alcoholism and obesity but stress has not been proven to cause cancer. The psychological effects of stress on the body of one who has been diagnosed with cancer has been found to cause a tumor to metastasize, having the ability to grow and spread throughout the body. According to the National Cancer Institute, the stress hormone norepinephrine could promote metastasis of cancer. Furthermore, stress may become overwhelming to the point of helplessness and may cause one to not seek treatment, follow medical advice or give up early in the treatment process. Emotional stress is also related to a person's ability to heal and manage disease and treatment positively. For example, studies have shown that stress management has been linked to less relapses therefore limiting growth.

Below are suggestions for cancer patients to cope with psychological stress according to National Cancer Institute:

> Training, education in relaxation, meditation or stress management.

> Counseling or talk therapy.

> Cancer education sessions.

> Social support in a group setting.

> Medications for depression and anxiety.

> Exercise.

Chapter Seven

Stress and Pain

Merriam-Webster defines pain as "the physical feeling caused by disease, injury, or something that hurts the body". The medical dictionary defines pain as "an unpleasant feeling that is conveyed to the brain by sensory neurons". It is important to note that the medical dictionary also states that "pain is more than a sensation, or the awareness of physical pain; it also includes perception, the subjective interpretation of the discomfort". This means that pain is specific to each individual, what may cause pain in someone, may not cause pain in another. Pain is specific to the way we think about it and how we believe it affects us. When one thinks of the mind and body connection, one can make the correlation between stress and pain. Thoughts and emotions often trigger physical reactions in the body. The mind and body do not function without one another. Emotional stress can affect the way one feels pain or the intensity of the pain. Research has proven that an important step to managing pain is managing stress. Chronic pain sufferers and individuals who have sustained injuries and diseases may reduce the effects of pain by lowering their stress levels. The brain is often working to identify and send pain signals, if one is chronically stressed, this may affect the brains ability to filter important signals and cause pain to be increased. According to a 2013 study, it was found that individuals with a smaller than average hippocampus are more vulnerable to stress. In relation to pain management, it was found that the reduction of stress decreases pain and prevents chronic pain (University of Montreal). The inability to manage stress and cope can enhance back, neck and shoulder pain due to a rise in cortisol levels. More research is needed in this area to determine the exact physiological causes of stress and the body's pain response, however pain threshold is proven to be managed and lowered by an effective stress management plan or utilizing relaxation techniques.

Link between Stress and Pain

Scientists have discovered there is a link to psychological stress and pain. Carnegie Mellon University conducted a study in 2012 and found that chronic psychological stress is associated with the body losing its ability to regulate the body's inflammatory response. The inability to regulate inflammation can also lead to disease progression and development of illnesses. The immune cells are unable to respond to hormonal signals that normally would regulation inflammation.

When the body is under stress it produces hormones that may increase muscle tension and pain sensitivity.

This may create physical symptoms or pain sensitivity in the body. For example, many people may recall a time when they were under stress or pressure and developed a headache. Most often, the head, neck and back often hold tension and pain due to stress and anxiety. This is an area that massage practitioners often focus on to relieve tension and pain in the muscles and body. Not only the head, neck and shoulders but our stomach is often an area where symptoms may appear during times of stress and anxiety. Ulcers may form and cause severe pain and other stomach problems in the body or digestive system. The stomach and bowels may ache or be upset or one may develop constipation or diarrhea and even nausea. All of these can become gastrointestinal problems such as GERD, Chrohn's disease and irritable bowel syndrome or IBS. Others while under stress may experience pain in the jaw or stiffness and grind their teeth which can lead to dental issues. Grinding teeth also called bruxism, can damage teeth or oral health complications if continuous. All of these symptoms may be due to stress and cause pain in the body. The various symptoms range from cognitive, physical, as well as behavioral when the body experiences stress.

Some results of long term stress or chronic stress on the mind and body are as follows:

- ➢ Personality disorders, depression and anxiety

- ➢ Heart attacks, stroke, high blood pressure and atherosclerosis

- ➢ Obesity or eating disorders

- ➢ Menstrual problems

- ➢ Sexual dysfunction - impotence and loss of desire

- ➢ Acne, psoriasis and hair loss

- ➢ Gastrointestinal issues- ulcers, IBS and GERD

All of these issues that manifest in the physical body and mind are directly result from unattended stress on the body, or chronic anxiety poorly managed or prevented.

Prevention is important and there are many ways to reduce and eliminate stress that assist in maintaining mental and physical health. We will discuss these prevention methods later in another chapter. Another way to view the effects of stress on the body in terms of pain is to think of a chain, the more weight and pressure put on the chain, the chain will eventually break under too much pressure. This is how the body works, the body is built to take care of itself, however the more pressure and stress put on the body, and the systems start to weaken just like links in a chain and breakdown leaving the body at risk for illness and disease.

According to the American Psychological Association (2014), stress affects the musculoskeletal system. The musculoskeletal system is made up of muscles, tendons, ligaments, bones, cartilage, joints and bursae. The body's way of preventing injury and pain is to tense up when stressed, muscle tension leaves the body when the stress is gone. Chronic stress may cause the muscles in the body to be in a constant state of tension which may trigger other harmful reactions in the body.

Chapter Eight

Stress Management

Stress management is about self-awareness, knowing what your sources of stress are, and creating strategies to cope or manage them effectively. Many of these strategies will involve changing daily routines such as diet, sleep, exercise, and relaxation. To maintain a healthy balance, this may require seeking medical help, creating a strong support system and learning new techniques to manage work, family and self-care.

According to the American Psychological Association (APA) in 2012, "only 37 percent of Americans feel they are actually doing an excellent or very good job of managing their stress". It is important to remember that stress is subjective and what may be stressful for one individual may not be stressful to someone else, the same applies to stress management. The key is to find what works best for your individual lifestyle and preference. Awareness and recognition of stress symptoms is important so that stressors can be identified and managed. Even small steps taken one day at a time can help to eliminate stress. Stress may be unavoidable completely, that is why healthy management is essential.

Simple Techniques to Offset Stress

Simple techniques may be used to manage stress daily. It may help to do tiny steps every day to make the process of overcoming stress seem less overwhelming or difficult. Here are some (not exhaustive) suggestions:

- ➢ Go for a daily walk.

- ➢ Take deep breaths in and out.

- ➢ Read something positive or inspiring.

- ➢ Take a long bath at the end of your day.

- ➢ Talk to friends and family.

- ➢ Listen to music.

- ➢ Laugh often and make time for fun.

- ➢ Learn how to say "No".

- ➢ Keep a stress journal.

- ➢ Spend some time outdoors in nature.

Breathing Exercises for Stress

Scientists and research has discovered many benefits to breathing exercises and focusing on controlled breathing. When the body is stressed and is disturbed by the release of stress hormones, stressors throw the nervous system out of balance. Focusing on calming the mind and body can be achieved through breathing which will produce the body's relaxation response. The relaxation response brings the nervous system back to a balanced state of equilibrium (homeostasis).

Many of the Eastern practices for mind and body health such as Yoga, Thai chi, and meditation focus the mind on breathing and relaxation. There are several breathing techniques to choose from and some may vary in their effectiveness depending on the individual. The importance about choosing a breathing technique is to choose one which triggers the body's relaxation response. The American Institute of Stress (AIS) lists two techniques to assist the mind and body connection to decrease the stress response:

> ➢ Quieting Response-Deep breathing and visualization for 6 seconds. *Smile*

inwardly using your eyes and mouth and

release the tension in your shoulders.

Imagine holes in the soles of your feet,

breath in while visualizing hot air flowing

through the holes upwards to legs,

abdomen and lastly lungs. Relax. When

exhaling, reverse the visualization; see the

air coming out of the holes in your feet.

Repeat if necessary to relax.

➢ Sudarshan Kriya or (SKY)-Series of
   breathing techniques that involve
   rhythmic breathing to harmonize the
   body, mind and emotions.

These techniques can relieve negative emotions
such as anger, frustration and depression. There

are a series of rhythmic exercises as well. For more information online visit artofliving.org.

The AIS has many helpful tools and breathing techniques, it is recommended to set aside anywhere from 5-10 minutes a day or more to practice the various techniques to de-stress and calm the mind and body. Benefits of deep breathing are linked to affect the heart, brain, digestion and immune system.

The simplest breathing technique for relaxation is to breathe in through the nose and exhale through the mouth, repeating this several times is proven to give oxygen to your brain and provide a calmer state. This can be done anywhere and for a short interval to achieve a

more relaxed state.

Chapter Nine

Stress and the Reproductive System

The Reproductive System supports the body's ability to create life and sustain the human population. The reproductive system consist of the male and female genitalia organs and the internal organs that produce hormones and substances needed for reproduction. While some may not understand the importance of the reproductive system, let's suppose in time that humans become limited in the reproduction process due to some unforeseen disease or plague, the human race becomes an endangered species. Stress can affect the body's ability to reproduce; therefore it is important to understand the impact on the reproductive organs. The reproductive system for both men and women is maintained by hormones.

Male Reproductive System

There are three main parts in the male reproductive system:

➤ Penis

➤ Scrotum

➤ Testes

For men, the reproductive system consists of the penis, scrotum and the testes which produce sperm. The penis is the organ used during sexual intercourse. The scrotum (sac) contains two testes (gonads) that are responsible for producing testosterone and sperm. The male hormone that is produced from the testes is called testosterone; this creates the cells in sperm necessary for fertilization. Semen is the fluid that carries the sperm for reproduction and is ejaculated out of the male during sexual intercourse. The penis is made up of pockets of erectile tissue that allow it to become filled with blood for an erection. An erection is related to blood flow regulated by the erectile tissue and penile arteries relaxing and contracting. Stress affects the male reproductive system in various ways. One of the ways that stress can harm the reproductive system is Erectile Dysfunction (ED).

In men, erectile dysfunction or a restriction of blood flow to sexual organs may cause inactivity and even more psychological stress. Impotence is common in males and can affect ejaculation and the ability to orgasm in both male and females. When a male is under stress, the blood flow may be restricted due to blood flowing to keep other organs such as the brain and the heart functioning properly, therefore hindering an erection. For example anxiety, depression and fear may prevent the brain from signaling the nervous system to maintain the proper levels required for an erection. Medical conditions such as vascular diseases that restrict blood flow may also prevent an erection. Diseases and conditions that affect the nervous system may also interfere with erections such as diabetes or alcoholism. The stress hormone cortisol may affect the levels of

testosterone produced which in turn affects

sexual desire. There are many causes that may

contribute to erectile dysfunction (ED), it is

important to seek medical assistance to

determine physiological or psychological causes.

Research has argued that both men and women

often feel ashamed or embarrassed about sexual

dysfunction and may be reluctant to seek

medical attention and treatment.

Female Reproductive System

There are three main parts in the female reproductive system:

- ➢ Vagina
- ➢ Uterus
- ➢ Ovaries

The female reproductive system consists of the vagina, uterus, and the ovaries. The female hormone produced from the ovaries is estrogen. Both estrogen and testosterone are essential to produce eggs and sperm for fertilization. When the body is functioning well and in good health, the production of both of the male and female hormones are automatically produced by both. When the body is under stress or prolonged periods of stress, infertility or sexual dysfunction may occur. This could be for men or women due to the stress hormone cortisol released in the body which may inhibit a man's sexual hormones and lower sperm count for males and reduce ovulation in females. Why does this occur one might ask? For starters, cortisol reduces desire for sexual activity because it decreases the reproductive hormones that are required for the fertilization process. So some individuals may not engage in sexual activity and chronic stress may also interfere with fertility and erections.

It is not uncommon for women who are under stress or chronically depressed to have irregular and painful menstruation periods. This may interfere with ovulation and the production of eggs and put women at higher risk for miscarriage. Pre-menstrual symptoms such as cramping, heavy bleeding, and fluid retention may worsen due to stress, cycles may even be prolonged or more frequent. Menopause may also cause women stress due to the fluctuation of hormones, mood swings, hot flashes and anxiety. Mental or emotional stress may cause the symptoms of menopause to be worse than normal.

Depression, unhealthy diet, lack of exercise and obesity are also causes of impotence or erectile dysfunction. One can see how the lifestyle choices and habits that are a result from stress mirror the same issues that cause sexual dysfunction.

Infertility

According to the U.S. National of Child and Human Development, the definition of infertility, (also called sterility) is "not being able to become pregnant after a year of trying". If a women gets pregnant but continues to have stillbirths or miscarriages, this is also known as infertility. After one year of unprotected sexual intercourse, 15 percent of couples are unable to become pregnant, third of the cases are attributed to women, another third to men and the rest attributed to both sexes. Infertility may be caused by physical, behavioral and environmental factors. The more frequent causes of male infertility are low or impaired sperm production, lifestyle or behavioral issues, or harmful environmental exposures. The frequent causes for female infertility are hormonal imbalance, reproductive organ dysfunctions, and behavior or environmental issues.

Stress is a risk factor for both men and women regarding fertility and is often treated by medication, surgery, and other assistive reproductive technologies. It is important to manage stress but if one is experiencing symptoms of sexual or reproductive dysfunction, it is even more important to seek medical help because often there are treatments and solutions that can reduce stress and the dysfunction causes.

Chapter Ten

Stress and Unemployment

Unemployment simply put, means not employed or without a job. The stress of unemployment can lead to many unfavorable outcomes. In addition to its physical fore-mentioned effects, stress can lead to declines in the well-being of spouses and to changes in family relationships and in outcomes for children.

Research dating back to the Great Depression found that men who experienced substantial financial loss became more irritable, tense, and explosive. Children often suffered as these fathers became more punitive and arbitrary in their parenting. Such paternal behavior, in turn, predicted temper tantrums, irritability, and negativism in children, especially boys, and moodiness, hypersensitivity, feelings of inadequacy and lowered aspirations in adolescent girls. Other studies have continued to find such a pathway from economic loss to father's behavior to child's well-being.

Depression has also been found among unemployed single mothers, and mothers who were more depressed more frequently punished their adolescent children. Frequently punished adolescent children, in turn, experienced increased distress and increased depressive symptoms of their own.

Unemployment may even impact decisions

about marriage and divorce. Unemployed or poor men are less likely to marry and more likely to divorce than men who are employed or who are more economically secure.

The impact of unemployment extends beyond individuals and families to communities and neighborhoods. High unemployment and poverty go hand in hand, and the characteristics of poor neighborhoods amplify the impact of unemployment. Inadequate and low-quality housing, underfunded schools, few recreational activities, restricted access to services and public transportation, limited opportunities for employment - all characteristics of poor neighborhoods - contribute to the social, economic, and political exclusion of individuals and communities, making it more difficult for people to return to work. In a six country study, increased risk of mortality was associated with higher neighborhood unemployment rates.

Unemployed workers also report less neighborhood belonging than those employed. Occupational networks are also impacted. Coworkers who have not lost their jobs may suffer from anxiety that they, too, will soon be fired, and from a heavier work load, as they must now take on the work once done by their former colleagues. Those who retain their jobs in the midst of downsizing may experience the comparable effects of physical and emotional

stress, just as workers who lose their jobs.

Chapter Eleven

When to get help

As discussed earlier, some stress is actually good (eustress) for life situations and give the body that boost of energy when needed. Eustress keeps the excitement in life and makes our lives fun and provides the necessary challenges to live with goals and purpose.

Eustress allows us to strive as human beings. This is healthy for living and without the positive stressors, the risk of becoming depressed and down about the meaning of life is high. It is unrealistic to experience a life without stress and stressful events, everyone experiences stress. The key is to maintain balance (homeostasis) between the normal stressors of life and the negative stressors that can cause systems to break down or slow their processes to maintain health. One of the requirements to maintain balance or homeostasis is to choose appropriate responses to stressors and develop a plan to manage stressors that includes prevention of chronic stress or prolonged stressors.

Acute stressors not managed properly or occurring frequently contribute to chronic stress. This causes stress overload. Stress overload is untreated chronic stress and can potentially harm almost every system in the body. Once stress is at the point of overload, the physiological risks of developing serious illnesses are high. It is at this point that an individual may feel like his or her life is out of control and unmanageable. The likelihood of poor eating/sleeping habits and depression may exist as well as alcohol/substance abuse to mitigate the feelings of being overwhelmed and loss of control.

Recognizing the warning signs of stress early is critical to avoid overload. It is easier to cope with stress before it gets to harmful in overload. Stress overload that keeps the body in a constant state of imbalance can cause damage to the brain, heart, respiratory and immune system which will make the management of stressors more difficult. If one is experiencing overload, overcoming stressors may still be possible, however more outside assistance (medical) and consistent efforts on behalf of the individual may be required to achieve balance again.

Seeking Help

Dealing with stress and managing the daily demands of life is difficult especially if one is trying to handle stressors alone. If stress is unmanageable or one is unable to detect what is causing the stress either psychologically or physically, it may be time to seek medical assistance. When all resources have been exhausted such as stress management techniques, close friends, family and clergy are not available or the body has been under chronic stress for a long period, seek medical support. There is nothing to be embarrassed or ashamed of, stress is a harmful disease that must be diagnosed and treated just like any other disease like diabetes or cancer. It is important to recognize the signs and seek help if necessary. Seeking help is wise and is necessary for selfcare when having problems.

It is important to seek immediate medical attention if the following exist:

- ➤ You are having thoughts of harming yourself or others.

- ➤ Stressors are frequent and regular, lasting weeks, months, or years.

- ➤ Work or school performance has declined.

- ➤ Abuse of alcohol, drugs and tobacco to relieve stress.

- ➤ Unable to accomplish daily tasks, routines.

- ➤ Are markedly withdrawn and sad for long periods.

- ➤ Experiencing irrational thoughts and behaviors.

- ➤ Significant weight loss or weight gain.

  - ➤ Significant changes in sleep

  patterns.

- ➤ Persistent pain and physical problems.

Reflection

Understanding stress, the body's response to stress both physically and mentally is complicated and may be a different experience for everyone. Each person is unique and how stress affects their life and the ability to cope may vary as well. It is not wise to compare your situation and circumstances to someone else as each individual's stress threshold and abilities are different, what may seem overwhelming to one person may be easier for another. Therefore seeking medical attention according to your own personal situation and judgment is necessary.

There are various stress management programs, clinics, helpful information online and medical solutions available for everyone. Many employers and insurance companies have stress treatment solutions and offer counseling to employees and customers. The most important thing is to recognize stress and seek appropriate solutions and treatment that work best for you.